RED SMOOTHIE DETOX FACTOR

35 Nourishing Red Smoothie Detox Recipes To Clean Your Gut, Help You Lose Weight And Feel Amazing In Under 30 Days!

By KATYA JOHANSSON

Copyright © 2016 By Katya Johansson.

All Rights Reserved.

Introduction

Red Smoothie Detox uncovered a detox control recipe that energizes weight reduction and thusly scrubs the assortment of harmful substances. Named as one of the main and most looked for after detox guide on the web, the author, guarantees planned clients of the nature of item.

It works in light of a hidden push to help people show signs of improvement comprehension of the detox procedure.

The aide all things considered is bespoke of individual detox needs, which implies it permits clients space to make a solicitation for a particular detox administration of their picking, either for blood, body, oral or hair detox.

The creator of the aide makes strong cases about the adequacy of the red smoothie detox variable, indicating at the way that it uncovers the missing "element" that guarantees the proficiency of the detoxification procedure. Recorded and properly clarified inside the aide are the four fixings: Maca, Vanilla, Cocoa and Chia. With the creator, expressing that her point is for the normal individual inspired by flushing out poisonous body substances would have the capacity to show signs of improvement.

Contents

1. Amazing Red Detox Smoothie — 1
2. Cleansing Red Smoothie — 2
3. Anti-Inflammatory Amazing Red Smoothie — 3
4. Red Fruit Smoothie — 4
5. Healthy Berry Red Smoothie — 5
6. Red Berry with Beet Smoothie — 6
7. Delicious Red Citrus Detox Smoothie — 7
8. Red Velvet Smoothie — 8
9. Red Antioxidant Tasty Smoothie — 9
10. Delicious Coco-Beet Smoothie — 10
11. Red Fruit Smoothie — 11
12. Beet Fruit Smoothie — 12
13. Amazing Spicy & Sweet Beet Smoothie — 13
14. Pink Tasty Smoothie — 14
15. Healthy Strawberry Kiwi Smoothie — 15
16. Berry Pie like Smoothie — 16
17. Creamy Red Velvet Smoothie — 17
18. Fired Red Smoothie — 18

19. Amazing Avocado Smoothie _____ 19

20. Beet Salad with Honey, Orange Vinaigrette _____ 20

21. Smoothie with Blueberries, Orange and Kale _____ 22

22. Healthy Berry Breakfast _____ 23

23. Strawberry with Kiwi Smoothie _____ 24

24. Watermelon Smoothie _____ 25

25. Berry Tasty Smoothie _____ 26

26. Soy Tasty Smoothie _____ 27

27. Healthy Berry Breakfast _____ 28

28. The Sicilian _____ 29

29. Amazing Detox _____ 30

30. Amazing Cranberry Cleanser _____ 31

31. Fat Flush Smoothie _____ 32

32. Amazing Breakfast smoothie _____ 33

33. Red Tasty Berry Smoothie _____ 34

34. Red Berry, Healthy Cabbage and Almond Smoothie __ 35

35. Amazing Berry and Beet Smoothie _____ 36

1. Amazing Red Detox Smoothie

Ingredients

- 1/2 cup crude red beets, cleaved
- 1 Tbsp cacao powder
- 1/3 cup raspberries crisp or solidified
- 1 cup water lemon water

Method

1. Mix all Ingredients until smooth and no pieces show up.
2. Present with a (re-useable) straw

2. Cleansing Red Smoothie

Ingredients

- bunch of crisp spinach
- 1/4 glass red beetroot, peeled
- 2 little apples (what's in season), quartered
- 1 medium banana, peeled
- 1 mandarin, peeled (ensure it has no pits)
- 1 cm bit of ginger
- juice of 1/2 major lemon (I utilized Meyer)
- 1/2 tsp cinnamon
- 1 TBSP chia seeds
- 1.5 to 2 mugs water
- Discretionary: more chia seeds to serve

Method

1. Hurl all to blender and rush until you get a rich, smooth consistency.

3. Anti-Inflammatory Amazing Red Smoothie

Ingredients

- 1 medium beet, peeled and cubed
- 2 cups strawberries, new or solidified
- 1/4 cup coconut oil, additional virgin
- 3 Medjool dates, set
- 1 cup apple cuts (discretionary)
- 1/2 cups any milk (I utilized unsweetened almond milk)

Method

Add all Ingredients to a rapid blender and procedure until extremely smooth, around 4-5 minutes. Serve instantly.

4. Red Fruit Smoothie

Ingredients

- 1/2 vast banana, cut into pieces
- 2 crisp strawberries, washed and cut
- 1/4 cup blueberries
- 1/2 glass milk
- 1 teaspoon vanilla concentrate
- 2 tablespoons vanilla yogurt
- 2 ice 3D shapes

Method

1. Place the banana pieces, strawberries, blueberries, milk, vanilla concentrate, yogurt, and ice 3D shapes in a blender. Mix until smooth.

5. Healthy Berry Red Smoothie

Ingredients

- 11/4 cups squeezed apple
- banana
- cup solidified strawberries
- cup solidified raspberries

Method

1. Add Ingredients to Four Side or Wild Side+ jar all together recorded and secure cover.
2. Select "Smoothie" or mix on a Medium velocity for 50-60 seconds.

6. Red Berry with Beet Smoothie

Ingredients

- glasses blended solidified red berries, for example, strawberries and raspberries
- 1 little red beet, peeled and meagerly cut
- 1 tablespoon crisp lemon juice
- 1 tablespoon honey
- 2 teaspoons foul virgin coconut oil

Method

1. Put the berries, 1/2 glass chilly water, beet, lemon juice, honey and coconut oil into a blender.
2. Mix on high until smooth, killing the blender and pushing down on the Ingredients with a spatula or wooden spoon as expected to help the mixing procedure. Add 1 to 2 tablespoons more water if necessary to conform consistency.

7. Delicious Red Citrus Detox Smoothie

Ingredients

- 1 cup beet greens
- 1/2 medium crude beet, cut into pieces
- 1/2 grapefruit, peeled + seeded
- 1/2 cup solidified pineapple pieces + more to taste
- 1/4 cup new cranberries
- Juice from 1/2 lemon
- Press of new squeezed orange
- 1 cup coconut water
- 1 tsp – 1 tbsp coconut oil
- Ice (discretionary)
- crude honey (discretionary)

Topping

: chia pudding, goji berries, crude pumpkin seeds, crude shelled hemp seeds

Method

1. Put all Ingredients in a rapid blender and mix on high until smooth.
2. Top with chia pudding, goji berries, pumpkin seeds and shelled hemp seeds.

8. Red Velvet Smoothie

Ingredients

- mugs new spinach
- 2 mugs coconut milk, unsweetened
- 2 mugs strawberries
- dates, set
- ¼ glass diced crude or cooked beets
- 1 tablespoon cacao powder
- ½ teaspoon vanilla concentrate (discretionary)
- Coconut whipped cream on top (discretionary)

Method

1. Mix spinach and coconut milk until smooth.
2. Include remaining Ingredients, and mix until smooth. Appreciate!

9. Red Antioxidant Tasty Smoothie

Ingredients

- 1 glass (250 ml) coconut water
- ½ pomegranate, seeds as it were
- 1 vast bunch of red grapes
- ½ glass (75 g) strawberries
- 1 bunch of ice

Method

1. Plan pomegranate by tailing this simple 3-stage, no-wreckage process from the Pomegranate Council, to demonstrate to you proper methodologies to de-seed a pomegranate.
2. Include all Ingredients into the blender and mix on high for 45 – 60 seconds until smooth.

10. Delicious Coco-Beet Smoothie

Ingredients

- 1 glass (250 ml) coconut water
- 1 cut of pineapple
- ½ glass strawberries
- 1/3 brilliant beet
- beet clears out
- little leaves of stevia
- 1 bunch of ice

Method

1. Expel external skin from pineapple.
2. Add all Ingredients to blender and mix on high for 45 – 60 seconds until smooth.

11. Red Fruit Smoothie

Ingredients

- 1 mugs seedless red grapes
- blood oranges, peeled
- 1 container solidified or crisp cranberries
- 1 pomegranate (seeds as it were)
- 1 container extremely frosty water
- Discretionary: sweetener of decision

Method

1. Put every one of the fixings in your blender and blend on rapid until very much joined.
2. Taste to check whether it is sufficiently sweet for you.

12. Beet Fruit Smoothie

Ingredients

- 1 glass (250 ml) coconut water
- ½ winged serpent natural product
- ½ banana (crisp or solidified)
- ¼ beet (beetroot)
- ½ lime, crushed
- 1 bunch of blended greens, for example, lettuce, arugula (rocket) and spinach
- 1 bunch of ice

Method

1. Peel the winged serpent products of the soil.
2. Include every one of the Ingredients into the blender and mix for 45 – 60 seconds until smooth.

13. Amazing Spicy & Sweet Beet Smoothie

Ingredients

- 1 cup (250 ml) coconut water
- 1/2 cup (55 g) fruits (crisp or solidified)
- 1/4 beet (beetroot)
- 1/2 stew pepper (discretionary)
- 1 bunch of ice

Method

1. Peel the beet and pit the fruits, if utilizing new.
2. Include every one of the Ingredients into the blender for 45 – 60 seconds until smooth.

14. Pink Tasty Smoothie

Ingredients

- 1/2 cup (50 g) red currants
- 1/2 glass (55 g) raspberries
- 1/2 banana
- 1 cut of pineapple (full circle cut)
- 1 glass (250 ml) coconut water
- 1 bunch of ice

Method

1. Peel the banana.
2. Include Ingredients into the blender and mix on high until smooth.

15. Healthy Strawberry Kiwi Smoothie

Ingredients

- 1/2 glasses (375 ml/12 oz) coconut water
- kiwi (kiwifruit)
- 1/2 glasses (225 g) solidified strawberries
- 1/2 solidified banana
- 1/4 avocado
- 1 tbsp crisp lime juice
- 1 tbsp maple syrup (discretionary for included sweetness)

Method

1. Peel kiwi and expel stem from strawberries.
2. Add all Ingredients to blender and blender on high for 45 – 60 seconds until smooth

16. Berry Pie like Smoothie

Ingredients

- 1 cup/125 g raspberries (new or solidified)
- 1 cup/125 g strawberries (new or solidified)
- tbsp goji berries
- 1 tbsp lucuma powder
- 1 cup/250 ml almond milk

Method

1. Include every one of the Ingredients into the blender.
2. Mix on high for 45 – 60 seconds and enhancement with additional berries to add a bite component if sought!

17. Creamy Red Velvet Smoothie

Ingredients

- 1/4 – 1/2 beet (beetroot)
- 1/2 avocado
- 1 tbsp cacao powder
- 1 tsp chia seeds
- 1/2 cup (125 ml) coconut drain or nut milk
- 1 cup (250 ml) water or coconut water
- 1 bunch of ice
- tsp of maple syrup or unadulterated honey
- dash of cinnamon (discretionary)

Method

1. Peel the beetroot – (discretionary – I do this for smoothies just) and scoop out the avocado tissue.
2. Put all Ingredients in blender.
3. Mix on high for 45 – 60 seconds until smooth.
4. Serve and appreciate.

18. Fired Red Smoothie

Ingredients

- 1 pomegranate
- tbsp goji berries
- 1 date
- 1/4 - 1/2 little beet (beetroot)
- 1/2 glasses (375 ml) coconut water (or coconut ice – solidified coconut ice 3D squares)

Method

1. Evacuate the pomegranate seeds – Follow this simple 3-stage, no-chaos process from the Pomegranate Council.
2. Peel the beet (beetroot).
3. Put all Ingredients in blender.
4. Mix on high for 45 – 60 seconds until smooth and pour on ice.

19. Amazing Avocado Smoothie

Ingredients

- 3/4 glass (125 g) raspberries new or solidified
- 1/2 cup (75 g) strawberries new or solidified
- 1/2 avocado
- 1 bunch arugula (rocket)
- 1 cup (250 ml) unsweetened almond or coconut milk
- 1 scoop unflavored pea or hemp protein, discretionary

Method

1. Consolidate Ingredients in blender.
2. Mix until smooth, around 60 – 90 seconds.
3. Serve and appreciate!

20. Beet Salad with Honey, Orange Vinaigrette

Ingredients

- glasses shredded crude red beets
- 1 shallot, peeled, finely slashed
- tablespoons red wine or balsamic vinegar (can likewise utilize a champagne vinegar)
- ½ orange or 1 tangerine
- 1 teaspoon honey
- tablespoons grapeseed oil (or canola)
- tablespoons additional virgin olive oil
- Ocean salt,
- Dark pepper

Method

1. Peel and mesh red beets (I utilized sustenance processor). Put aside.
2. Pizzazz the citrus. Put aside.
3. In little sustenance processor, place shallot, a crush of citrus, honey and vinegar. Blend well. Include both oils. Keep on mixing. Season with salt and pepper.
4. Hurl beets the vinaigrette. (You won't utilize it all, this ought to be sufficient for 4 measures of beets on

the off chance that you need to twofold formula. Use remaining dressing for another plate of mixed greens).
5   Hurl with the greater part of citrus pizzazz, sparing some for trimming.
6   You can serve now or refrigerate and serve later.

21. Smoothie with Blueberries, Orange and Kale

Ingredients

- 1 orange, peeled
- 1 bunch kale
- 1 bunch spinach
- 1 carrot
- 1 apple, cut down the middle, center and seeds evacuated
- measures of blueberries
- 1 little crude red beet, peeled
- ½ glass water
- 1 glass ice

Method

1. Place Ingredients in Vitamix, and hit the smoothie catch, or blend until every one of the Ingredients are pounded into a smoothie. Include more water if vital.

22. Healthy Berry Breakfast

Ingredients

- 1 c solidified unsweetened raspberries
- ¾ c chilled unsweetened almond or rice milk
- ¼ c solidified set unsweetened fruits or raspberries
- 1½ Tbsp honey
- tsp finely ground crisp ginger
- 1 tsp ground flaxseed
- tsp crisp lemon juice

Method

1. Join all Ingredients in blender, adding lemon juice to taste. Puree until smooth.
2. Fill 2 chilled glasses.

23. Strawberry with Kiwi Smoothie

Ingredients

- 1¼ c cool apple
- 1 ready banana, cut
- 1 kiwifruit, cut
- solidified strawberries
- 1½ tsp honey

Method

1. Join the juice, banana, kiwifruit, strawberries, and honey. Mix until smooth.

24. Watermelon Smoothie

Ingredients

- c cleaved watermelon
- ¼ c sans fat milk
- 1 c ice

Method

1. Join the watermelon and drain, and mix for 15 seconds, or until smooth.
2. Include the ice, and mix 20 seconds longer, or to your wanted consistency. Include more ice, if necessary, and mix for 10 seconds

25. Berry Tasty Smoothie

Ingredients

- 1½ c cleaved strawberries
- 1 c blueberries
- ½ c raspberries
- Tbsp honey
- 1 tsp new lemon juice
- ½ c ice blocks

Method

Mix all Ingredients and blend

26. Soy Tasty Smoothie

Ingredients

- 1 c calcium-invigorated vanilla soy milk
- ½ c solidified blueberries
- ½ c corn drops oat
- 1 solidified banana, cut

Method

1. Join the milk, blueberries, oat, and banana in a blender for 20 seconds.
2. Scratch down the sides and mix for an extra 15 seconds.

27. Healthy Berry Breakfast

Ingredients

- 1 glass solidified unsweetened raspberries
- 3/4 glass chilled unsweetened almond or rice milk
- 1/4 glass solidified set unsweetened fruits or raspberries
- 1/2 Tbsp honey
- tsp finely ground crisp ginger
- 1 tsp ground flaxseed
- 1-2 tsp crisp lemon juice

Method

1. Join all Ingredients in blender, adding lemon juice to taste.

28. The Sicilian

Ingredients

- carrots
- substantial tomatoes
- red chime peppers
- cloves garlic
- stalks celery
- 1 cup watercress
- 1 cup approximately stuffed spinach
- 1 red jalapeño, seeded (discretionary)

Method

1. WASH and prepare all Ingredients.
2. Squeeze all Ingredients.

29. Amazing Detox

Ingredients

- 1 tablespoon of cacao powder
- tablespoons of hemp seeds
- 4-5 red endive takes off
- green stevia
- ¼ measure of natural new or solidified dull red fruits
- 8-12 oz unadulterated water

Method

Mix all Ingredients and blend

30. Amazing Cranberry Cleanser

Ingredients

- ½ cup cranberries
- 1 huge celery stalk
- 1 cucumber
- 1 apple
- 1 pear
- spinach

Method

1   Mix all Ingredients and blend.

31. Fat Flush Smoothie

Ingredients

- 1 medium natural red beet
- medium natural carrots
- 1 natural radish
- natural garlic cloves
- parsley

Method

1. Mix all Ingredients and blend.

32. Amazing Breakfast smoothie

Ingredients

- 1 little ready banana
- around 140g blackberries, blueberries, raspberries or strawberries
- (then again utilize a blend), in addition to additional to serve
- squeezed apple or mineral water, discretionary
- runny honey

Method

1. Cut the banana into your blender or sustenance processor and include your preferred berries. Whizz until smooth.
2. With the sharp edges humming, pour in juice or water to make the consistency you like. Hurl a couple of additional organic products on top, shower with honey and serve.

33. Red Tasty Berry Smoothie

Ingredients

- 350g new strawberries, slashed
- 1 cup crisp raspberries or solidified raspberries
- 1/2 cups (around 180g) solidified yogurt
- 1 cup milk
- 1/3 cup SPLENDA

Method

1. Place strawberries, raspberries, solidified yogurt, milk and SPLENDA® in a blender. Mix until smooth. Fill glasses. Serve.

34. Red Berry, Healthy Cabbage and Almond Smoothie

Ingredients

- ½ glass newly crushed squeezed orange
- 1 glass blended solidified berries, ideally with a few fruits incorporated in with the general mish-mash
- ½ glass sliced red cabbage (50 grams)
- 1 teaspoon honey
- 1 teaspoon cinnamon
- or 3 drops almond separate (around 1/8 teaspoon)
- almonds or 2 teaspoons crude almond margarine
- ice solid shapes

Method

1. Put the majority of the Ingredients in a blender and mix for 1 min.
2. Fill a glass, trim with an orange cut and appreciate.

35. Amazing Berry and Beet Smoothie

Ingredients

- ½ cup crisply pressed squeezed orange
- 1 cup blended solidified berries or blueberries
- tablespoons granola
- 1 cup diced beet, either crude or cooked (50 grams)
- ¼ cup plain low-fat yogurt or low-fat coconut milk
- 1 teaspoon honey or agave syrup
- or 3 ice 3D shapes
- cut orange for embellishment (discretionary)

Method

1. Put the greater part of the Ingredients in a blender and mix for 1 min.
2. Fill a glass, trim with an orange cut and appreciate

Printed in Great Britain
by Amazon